NUMBER 664

THE ENGLISH EXPERIENCE

ITS RECORD IN EARLY PRINTED BOOKS
PUBLISHED IN FACSIMILE

(RICHARD HAWES)

THE POORE-MANS PLASTER-BOX

LONDON, 1634

WALTER J. JOHNSON, INC.
THEATRUM ORBIS TERRARUM, LTD.
AMSTERDAM 1974 NORWOOD, N.J.

The publishers acknowledge their gratitude to the Dean and Chapter of Peterborough Cathedral for their permission to reproduce the Library's copy, Classmark: Pet.G.21(3); and to the Trustees of the British Museum for their permission to reproduce pages B_2 v and F_3 v from the Library's copy, Shelfmark: 1038.G.42

S.T.C. No. 12942

Collation: A-F^4

Published in 1974 by

Theatrum Orbis Terrarum, Ltd.
O.Z. Voorburgwal 85, Amsterdam

&

Walter J. Johnson, Inc.
355 Chestnut Street
Norwood, New Jersey
07648

Printed in the Netherlands

ISBN 90 221 0664 0

Library of Congress Catalog Card Number:
74-80183

THE POORE-MANS PLASTER-BOX.

Furnished with diverse Excellent Remedies for sudden mischances, and usuall infirmities, which happen to Men, Women, and Children in this Age.

Whereunto is added certaine directions, whereby a man may know by what meanes a person (being found dead) came by his Death. Very fitting to be knowne of all such as are called to be Iurars upon Life and Death.

Published for the common good of all such *as stand in need, at the request of some well* disposed persons.

LONDON,
Printed by *Tho. Cotes*, for *Francis Grove*, and are to be sold at his shop upon Snow-hill, neere the Sarasens head.
1634.

THE POORE MANS *PLASTER-BOX,*

Furnished with divers excellent Remedies, for suddaine mischances, and usuall infirmities which happen to Men, Women, and Children in this Age.

For a small wound or hurt with Sword, Knife, Axe, or any other edge Toole.

My full intent and desire is to give direction to the poore and plaine people, such as cannot (for their remote living) get a Chirurgion, or else (dwelling where they may be had) want meanes to pay them for their paines; such people when they have any wound that is superficiall, (I meane which is not very deepe) whether it be done with Sword, Knife, Axe, Sithe, or Sickle, it makes no matter. Let them ioyne the lippes of the wound together so even as they can, and beate the white of an Egge with a little salt, and apply it with fine Flax or Lint made of an old cleane cloath, and

 roule

roule it so neately as you can. The next day open it and apply one of those wound-salves mentioned in this Booke, or else you may take sallet Oyle and a little Suggar, and dip Lint therein, and apply it.

Or take Mouse-eare and pouder it, and strew it in a greene wound, and it will heale it.

Also wilde Tansie chopt small, one handfull, Egs two; mingle them and fry them with sweet butter well washed from the salt, then strayne them, and it will be a good salve for greene wounds.

Or take Horse-taile or shave grasse and pouder it, and it will ioyne greene woands and heale them.

Brugle or Prunel strained and laid on a wound doth heale it.

Or Vervaine stamped with Honny and laid on as a plaster, healeth a wound or old soare in short time.

Comfry is a hearbe knowne to most people, take the leaves thereof and bruise them, and lay them on the wound and it will heale it. It is of such vertue that if the leaves be boyled in white wine and water, or water alone, (for neede) and put Honny therein, and drinke it morning and evening, it heales all hurts and bruses inwardly.

A good Plaster for greene wounds.

Take one pound of sheepes Suit, of Bittony, Millfoyle, and Scabious, of each one handfull: of sweet Butter without Salt halfe a pound; beate all these together in a Morter, and let them stand seaven dayes in a moyst place till they be mouley; then boyle them and let them be well strayned, then cut halfe a pound of Wax in small peeces, and Rosin as much, boyle them with the strained Iuices, and you have a good and needefulll plaine Plaster; use it boldly, and you shall find it will performe what was promised.

A good Vngnent for wounds.

Take Turpentine one ounce, oyle of Roses foure spoone-

fulls,

fulls, two yolkes of new laid Egges, mingle all these together and apply it on Lint, and over it lay the former Plaster.

But if it be for a wound where the flesh is brused, then lay it thicke on with fine Flax, and over it the whites of the Egges mingled with oyle of Roses, and roule it gently up.

A good cooling Plaster for greene wounds.

Take Ceruse three ounces, and sallet Oyle one pint, boyle them till it be reasonable thicke, and then add to it two ounces of yellow wax, so have you a good Plaster.

An Vnguent for wounds.

Take Turpentine of Venice two ounces, Honny of Roses one ounce, Barly meale halfe an ounce, then mingle them, and if it be too thicke, adde a little oyle to it and use it.

A good Vnguent for brused wounds.

Take Rosin, Pitch, and Wax of each two ounces, of sallet Oyle one pint, boyle them, and you shall have a good blacke oyntment.

An excellent Balsome for wounds.

Take sallet Oyle one pint, Wheate purged from the huskes and beaten, two ounces; put your Oyle and Wheate together, then take S. Iohns wort, valerian, and Carduus Benedictus, of each one ounce; infuse them in one pint of white wine eight houres, then put your Oyle and wine together, and let them boyle till the oyle have consumed the wine; then straine it and adde to the liquor foure ounces of good Turpentine, and let it boyle a little on a gentle fire, and you shall have a good Balsome, which you must use warme, and use a Plaster over it if you will; if not, dip a cloth in the Balsame, and lay it over the wound as you would a Plaster.

Another good Oyle for wounds.

Take oyle Olive halfe a pint, gum Elemny one ounce, Aqua vitæ thrée sponefulls; boyle them to the consumption of the Aqua vitæ, and you shall have an oyle to cure all wounds.

Sometimes the wound about the edges, and round about the wound, is very much inflamed and red, so that the patient cannot take any rest day or night; if it be in the beginning, use oyle of Roses thereto, and over all apply a linnen cloth, wet in one part of vinegar and two parts of faire water; or make this oyntment and lay it thereon:

Vnguent.

Take oyle of Roses one pint, Ceruse finely beaten two ounces, Camphore one quarter of an ounce; mingle them in a stone Mortar till it come to a perfect bodie, and you shall have a good cooling salve.

A Poultis for the same.

Take Mallowes, and Checkwéede, one handfull of each, bruise them small and boyle them in Cowes milke, with a little Barly meale, and put some oyle of Roses to it, and apply it warme.

Many times there growes a proud flesh in the wound which must be taken away ere that the wound will heale; to doe this take allome and burne it on a Tyle, and then pouder it and strew of the pouder on the proud flesh. Also you may use a red pouder which you may buy at the Apothecaries, but you had best to apply it with the burnt Allome; mingle them together, and it will worke the better.

Also you may take gréene Copperasse, and burne it in a pot till it be white and use it; it will doe its worke well, but it will worke painefully: but if you mingle some of these pouders with some unguent above written, it will worke the gentlier.

I would wish you, if you have any neighbour that hath skill in Chirurgery, to take his counsell in this case; for though the advise of many simple and pratling women, many honest people have béene spoyled, therefore take no such advise.

For bleeding of a wound.

If a wound bléed much, take the white of an Egge and some milldust, mingle them and lay it on with Flax or Lint, and binde it fast, and it will stop the bléeding; it hath béene often tryed and never failed.

Or if you be in the field that you can have none of these things at hand, then doe thus, it is both easie and certaine. Take of the Mosse that growes at the roote of an Oaken Trée, and lay it on the wound, and binde it close, and it will stop the blood.

Also take old and cleane linnen, burne it as you doe Tinder to strike fire with, and lay it on the wound, and it will stop the blood. These two last remedies I have séene used in the warres, when nothing could be gotten nor any Chirurgion was by to helpe the wounded men.

That wholesome Hearbe Sage stamped and layd to a wound, will stanch the blood.

The like doth Hearb-Robert, Pinckneedle, or Cranes-bill; it groweth commonly in hedges, bruise them and lay them on the wound.

Cinque-foyle or fiveleaved grasse doth the like, also Lysimachia or Lousestrife hath the same vertue.

For bleeding at the nose.

I have many times séene men bléede so fearefully at the nose, that unlesse there had béene present helpe, the parties had dyed; yet by these medicines and helpes following they were presently recovered.

Let the party lye on his backe, and let him have a wet cloth to receive the blood in, that his cloathes may be kept cleane: then bathe his Temples with cold water, and lay a double napkin wet in water and vinegar in his necke, and

hold

hold your two fourefingers hard on his Temples, and tell him also that it is stanched, though it bleede still; for that will worke strangely on his imagination as I have often found, so that he will gather strength suddainly, and the bleeding will cease.

I have found good successe by applying a cloth (wet in vineger and water) to the privy members; also by binding of the Arme on the same side with a garter, as the Chirurgions doe when they will let one blood: but you must not keepe it so bound longer than you may tell forty, but loose it and bind it againe; so doing till you finde that the blood is diverted, and stayd.

A pretty way to stanch bleeding at the Nose.

If the party bleede on the right side, then bow downe the little finger of the patient on the right side; if the patient bleed at the left nostrill, then bend the little finger of the left hand. I received this as a truth from a friend, if you prove it, you can receive no hurt by it.

Another remedy for bleeding at the Nose which hath helped divers to my knowledge.

Take Aloes one ounce, Mill dust, haires of a hare cut very small, whites of Egges, of each sufficient; take fine Flax and wet in it; when it hath beene well mingled, then make them pyramid-like, and put one of them into the nose that bleeds. I knew a woman of good fashion, who told me when shee was 16. yeares of age shee was taken with a great bleeding at the nose; this Flux of blood notwithstanding all the counsell of Physitians and of Chirurgions dured for the space of 48. houres, so that she was so weake that they expected her departure out of this life. An old woman comming in amongst other women and seeing her lye in that pittifull case, said that if Mugwort were applyed to the soles of her feete, questionlesse the bleeding would stay. In briefe, Mugwort was applyed, and she was suddainly helped. Thus much for bleeding at the nose, an accident by which many have lost their lives: but use these

remedies

remedies that I have set downe, and with Gods helpe you shall be able to helpe both your selfe and your friends.

Of wounds comming by biting of beasts.

The biting of madde dogges brings many times great danger, and for want of knowledge many dye of it, twelve Moneths after, as may be séene daily; if therefore any one be bitten, enquire whether the beast were madde or not; if the dogge or other beast that bit were not mad, then so much the better, and you néede feare the lesse.

If the wound be little, wash it with Vinegar and Honny; then lay some Treacle to it mingled with Turpentine and Butter, or else Garlicke and Onions stamped with Butter.

If the dogge were mad then take Treacle and wine, and rub the soare till it bléede, then apply Lint dipt therein, and over it Garlicke or Onions stamped and mingled; doe this seaven dayes together, and then apply other salves wherewith you cure wounds withall.

It were good that the partie so bitten should take somethinginwardly to defend the heart, for the which take of Venice Treacle the eight part of an ounce with some swéet wine; but if you have none, then take stale béere, mingle them and make it warme, and let the patient drinke it off and sweat after it.

This Venice Treacle you may buy at the Apothecaries; it is of such rare worth, that I could wish that every countrey man had of it in his house, the vertues are many, some of which I will set downe in these few words.

Venice Treacle

Doth cure all paines of the head in man or woman that comes through cold it is excellent good for all that are heavy hearted and fearefull, for those that have the falling sicknesse or any defluxion that procéedes from a cold cause, it helpeth the toothach and the falling of the pallat, if the place where the paine is be touched with it, and a plaster layd on the temple from whence the Flux commeth; it is good for the Squinancie, and helpes the dead palsie in the beginning; it is good for the paine of the stomacke, spitting of blood, for the griping of the belly and the bloody Flux; it helpeth the Crampe and those that are taken with Convulsions, which is drawing of the mouth and other members on the one side.

It breakes the stone, causeth the monethly termes, and destroyeth all infirmities of the wombe.

It is good for the Gout, Sciatica and paines of the Hips; but principally it is given for a helpe against poyson: it helpeth exceedingly against the bitings of mad Dogges or any other living thing, whether it be inwardly applied or outwardly on the wound, it helpeth those that are troubled with the quartan Ague, being taken a little before the fit commeth. I use to give it for the Ague with Carduus Benedictus water; iust when that they feele the fit comming let them take it and so sweate after it, it never yet failed me in this.

Of falls and bruses.

Often times it chanceth that many men in building fall from off the house, and many times lye as though they were dead with the paine thereof.

Also in felling of Trees men are soare brused, and not having remedy for them, they often perish for want of health: if such a misfortune come to thy friends or servants, doe as I shall direct thee, and feare not to doe much good with little charges.

If the partie falne lye without mooving as one dead, to know whether he be dead or not, doe this. Stop his nostrills and lay a feather or a little wooll on his mouth, and if there be any breath in him, they will stirre; If then that there is life in the partie, put a little Pepper in his nose to make him sneese: and if he doe bleed with sneesing, it is the better.

If you can get any to doe it, let him blood in the arme; my

reason

reason is this: the blood with the fall is fled inwardly to the heart, and lyes there in such quantity, that unlesse it be diverted by opening a veine, it is in danger to putrifie and corrupt the inward parts, and so occasions death.

If the bruise be on any part of the body (I meane under the head) annoint it with oyle of Roses, or give him some hot comfortable drinke to make him sweate, as good Muskadine, old Sacke, or Sacke and sallet Oyle; or Treacle and Carduus-water, and apply this outwardly.

A Poultis for bruises.

Take Cammomile, Wormewood, of each one handfull, red Rose leaves halfe a handfull, Barly meale one handfull, boyle them soft in water, and put fresh butter or oyle of Roses to it, and lay it hot on the place that is hurt, and cover him warme.

Wine Vineger and Sugar given to drinke is good, for it prevents all putrifaction and rottennesse, also if it be a little bruise, apply a cloth that is well wet in water and salt, for it is good.

A most excellent easy meanes for those that are hurt by falls or bruised: it is often approved and found good to my knowledge.

Take a Weathers skinne so soone as it is fleade off, and strew it with fine salt, and lap the patient so falne therein, but annoint him first with Oyle of Roses, and so let him sweate.

Then for inward meanes give him this drinke hot.

A drinke for bruises.

Take Plantaine leaves, and S. Iohns wort, Bittonny, Tansy, five leaved grasse, Colts foote, of each halfe a handfull, sweet Margeram, and Sage one handfull: stampe them and boyle them in thrée quartes of white wine, but if you haue no white wine, then boyle them in running water, add to it Honny, and boyle away the third part of it, then straine it and drinke thereof warme, morning and euening. Probatum est.

Wild-Sage boiled in white wine or in water with Honny is excellent for all falls or bruises.

Likewise Pellitory of Spaine cald in English Masterwort, boiled in wine, or water and Hony, is very good for the same.

A Poultis for blowes or stroakes.

Take Barrowes grease, Bran of Wheate, Fenegreke meale, Honny and wine, séeth all together and apply it to the bruise or stripe; it helpeth with spéed and giueth ease.

There is in Ireland a certaine spring that sendeth forth a muddy or fat water, this water through the heate of the Sun becommeth hard as a stone, and is of a darke blew like our Salte, and it is called Irish Slate: this Slate being scraped with a knife and drunke in Béere, Oyle or Wine, is good for all bruises, falls and also for the loosenesse of the belly.

A good remedy for a poore man.

If the man faln or bruised be so poore that he hath no bed to sweat in, then annoynt him with this following, and set him for to sweat in horse dung up to the chin, and couer his head with hay, this is so good meanes as may be used, but it is neither cleanly, nor chargeable.

The Oyntment.

Take a pound of swéete butter, put it in a frying pan, then take of parsly, and mosse, of each one handfull of Rew or hearbegrace, halfe a handful. chop them small and fry them in the butter till that the hearbes be dry, then straine them and annoint the partie falne therewith.

If that the patient, be falne on his backe that there is great paine, and yet no bone broken or out of Joynt, then doe thus.

Take halfe a pecke of Bran, boyle it in water that it be almost dry: then put to it two pound of Butter and stirre it well, then put it in a trough and let the man hurt lye on his backe therein.

Doe thus three times the day, and when it is cold renew it with hot Bran out of the kettle.

Then annoint him with Dialthea, or Spermaceti, or else one of the former Oyntments.

To drive away setled or blacke blood.

Take hard white Sope, commonly called Castle-Sope, cut it in small peeces; take of this Sope foure ounces, of unguentum Dialthea two ounces, of the best Aqua vitæ one quarter of a pint, melt them and annoint it twise a day.

A drinke for a poore man that is bruised.

Take earthwormes dryed, and oaken coales beaten, infuse these in Vinegar foure houres, then straine them and adde to it of Madder foure graines, warme it and drinke it.

For one that is beaten on the face that it is blacke and blew.

Take the iuce of wilde Saffran roote, and annoint it, or the iuce of Solamons Seale, Vng: Album, and the white of an egge, mingle them and annoint it in the morning, evening, and at noone.

This is approved for blacke Eyes.

Take the roote of blew flower Deluce, beate it with red rose water, then lay betweene a linnen Cloth and apply it to te the eyes, this never failes.

An Oyntment to soften all hard lumps, swellings, and Bruises, in any part of the Body; whether it cometh of inward or outward cause.

Take Mallow rootes one pound, Lint-seed halfe a pound. Cut your rootes, and bruise your seedes then steepe them in a pottle of water three dayes: at the three dayes end seeth them till the water be as a Slyme, then take one pint thereof, and mingle it with Hens grease, Goose grease, and Neates-foote oyle, of each halfe a pint; boyle them till the watrish part be consumed, then ad Waxe six ounces, Rosyn three ounces, and of Turpentine one ounce: let them boyle a little; and when you take them off mingle them in a morter till it be cold, and reserue it to your use.

For Deafenesse and paine in the Eares.

Many times poore men (that want the helpe of a Physition) by the want of means are troubled with deafenes and paine in the Eares: it cometh many times through cold, or by grosse humors stopping of the eares, or by an Impostum, or els some thing falne into the eare; those that are so troubled speake very low, and are troubled in their Sleepe.

In a Sun-shyning day looke in his eare to see the occasion of his paine, if any thing be falne into it, seeke to get it out, with some small Instrument: or doe this, let one person, or other blow into the eare so strongly as possible he can, and that a pretty space, then on a suddain let him sucke so strongly as he can: this is a good way to get any stone, graine, or any other thing out of the Eare.

For a Worme or Fly got in the Eare.

Put therein a drop of oyle of Wormewood, or the Juce of nut-rindes, or peach leaves, or doe this.

Take

Take a ripe Apple of good savour, cut it in two, and hollow it that the eare may come into it: apply this warme when you goe to bed, and in the morning you shall finde the worme dead in the Apple.

For Singing, or Piping in the Eares.

Put oyle of Hempseede warme into the eare, and stop it with sheeps wo ll, and let the Patient leape and use exercise, then lye downe on the side that he is payned, to see if any thing will run out.

To restore Hearing.

Stampe Earth-wormes, Emets egges, and the leaves of heartgrace; boyle these in Sallet oyle, and let one drop fall into the eare warme.

For one that is Deafe.

Take Rosemary and Rew, of each, halfe a handful: Chop them and boyle them in vineger, when that they are boyled, take a funnell that will fit the mouth of the pipkin, wherein the hearbes were boyled, cover it with the funnell and receive the fume into the eare, then put in a drop or two of oyle of bitter Almonds, and let him sweate after it.

Take greene Ash and put it into the fire, it will drop forth a liquor: this save and put into the eares that are payned, and it will cease the paine.

This is good for all paines in the Head, and for Deafenes.

Take Sallet oyle, Scalion seed, and the blades of leekes, with Wormewood and Rosemary, boyle these, and being strayned put one drop into thy eare, then stop it and lye not on the same side in sixe houres after

Another

Another.

Take the fat of an Ecle roasted, take an Onyon and Sengreene that groweth on the Tiles, beate all these together and straine it, and put thereof into the eare warm, and it will take away deafenesse.

Against all Diseases that afflict the Eyes.

There are many diseases incident to the Eyes, and they procéed of divers causes; they are written of at large in sundry bookes of learned men: and are not to be understood of every meane capacity, therefore I will passe over the causes, and for the signes, they are apparent enough, therfore I will set downe sundry approoved remedies for them.

To draw backe the humores that offend the Eyes.

Take leaven, figges, and mustardséed, beate these into a paste, and put to them a little vineger, and lay as much behinde in the necke as a five shilling péece of silver, this will draw a blister in one night, the next day cut the blister and lay to it a Colewoorte leafe, and it will draw it and heale it, this is safe and workes without danger.

A Plaster to stop the Reume.

Take Gum Elemny, and make a plaster on a little velvit or leather, and apply it to the Temples, and it will stay the Reume, that floweth to them.

Also take white frankensence and make a plaster, it will doe the like.

For hot Running Eyes,

Take an Apple, cald a Pomewater, boyle it in running water, then take of the pap and mingle it with a little white bread

bread crum that is soaked in a womans milke that gives a man Child sucke, put of this betwixt a fine linnen cloth and lay it to your eyes when that you goe to bed, and you shall finde great ease therein, this is without danger, and found perfect good.

For a pearle growing in the Eye.

Take ground Ivye, put some white wine thereto and stampe it, then straine it and put one drop into the sore Eye, morning and evening, and it will cure it without faile.

Another for the same.

Take the white of an egge, and the Juce of Perritory of the wall, beat them well together, and scame them: then put thereof into the Eye, and it will helpe it by Gods assistance.

Others for Red and blood-shotten Eyes.

Take new cheese often washed in faire water, beate it with the white of an egge and apply it to the eye, this is approved.

Take white Suggar-Candy, beate it very fine and put some of it into the eie, this is a secret, that hath holpen many.

Take the gaule of a Partridge, put some into the Eyes, and it will helpe the dimnesse of the sight.

The same doth the gaule of a Turtle dove, or the blood of a house dove.

The Juce of checkweed hath the same vertue.

An excellent water for soare Eyes, and to cleere the Sight.

Take foure sponefuls of white rose water, white Copperis, as much as a pease, ginger pared full as much, three Cloves: let these stand three houres in a beere glasse and with a feather scame off that which doth arise, then straine it and keep it in a viall, close stopped, and drop therof into your eye when you go to bed.

A salve for Red and running eyes.

Take fine powder of Tutty, foure parts; May butter three parts,

parts, Oyle of roses, two parts; melt these and mingle the powder till it be cold, and anoynt your Eyes therewith.

For the Tooth-ach many approoved Remedies.

The Tooth-ach, is a paine wherewith many people are much troubled, and it is a paine (being not mortall) the greatest of all other.

The cause proceedeth from the Sinewes, being very hot, or very cold, or else a great quantity of humors falling from the head to the gummes.

The signes are expressed by the patients grievous complaint, therefore I will set downe some remedies that I know are approved, and will give ease to the poore Patient.

A plaster for the Temples to stay the humour that falles on the Gummes.

Take Dragons blood, and pouder it, then mingle it with the white of an egge, and apply it to the Temples on both sides.

An excellent Oyle for the teeth, which hath helped many to my knowledge.

Take a sheete of white paper, teare it in small peeces, and burne it in a pewter dish, and there will come an oyle from it, with this oyle touch the aking tooth, or if it be hollow stop it with some of this oyle, it cureth it presently and is quickly gotten.

Another.

A learned and worthy Chirurgion on a time was grievously troubled with the Toothach, he used all the meanes, that he could thinke on for ease, but he found none; an old woman, coming to his house by chance and seeing him so payned, bid him to take a Clove of garlick and roast it, and lay it to his payned tooth; he did so, and was presently eased,

thus

thus Ambrose of Paris, sets down in his booke of Chirurgery.

Another.

Take salt mixt with dow, and bake it against the fire, and so laide on the Tooth easeth it presently.

Another.

When thou art troubled with the Tooth-ach, take good Aqua vitæ, and snuff up a little into the nostrill of the same side wherin you are payned, and that will ease you.

Also take good Methridate and rub your gummes where you are payned, and that will helpe presently.

Another.

Boyle henbane roote in vineger, and take of the vinegar and hold it in your mouth, and that doth ease it.

Boyle Coliquintida in vineger and hold it in your mouth, it helpeth.

To breake an hollow Tooth.

Fill the Tooth with Crowes dung, and it breakes the Tooth, and ceaseth the payne.

Take the roote of Pellitory of Spaine, and hold it in your mouth on the same side, and it helpeth without faile.

Pepper, Salt, and Garlick, beaten and put in a cloath and held in the mouth, is very good.

For an hollow Tooth.

Fill the Tooth with Treakle, and then take a sharpe stick of an Ash and burne it in the fire, and whilst it is lighted put it in the hollownesse of the Tooth, and it will leave aking.

But the best thing that you can do for a tooth that is hollow, is to plucke it out, or else it will be ever painefull, and corrupt your other teeth: but take heed that you meete with one that is expert in tooth drawing, least he break the Jaw, or pul forth a wrong tooth, as it once happened to a poore man that would have a Tooth drawne.

Merry tales sometimes easeth paine, and I know the Tothach is painefull : if it would ease you I care not much to tell you a tale of a Tooth-drawer.

A good Tooth-drawer.

In a Country village there dwelt a Tooth-drawer which was so famous in his Art that he was sought after farre and neere: this Tooth-drawer had a lusty young man to his servant, who had seene many Teeth drawne by his master, (with an Instrument, cald a Pellican, which will draw two teeth at one time unlesse it be skillfully handled.)yet never had he drawne any, which made him resolve that the next that came to have a Tooth drawne in his masters absence, he would venture on him. It chanced that a simple plaine man came on a day(when his master was at dinner) to have a tooth drawne,my yong Barber was glad of that, and bid him sit downe : and to worke he went with him with a Pellican, but see how it chanced, he for want of skill set the Pellican so that with his lubbers strength he drew out two of his sound teeth, and left the rotten in his head.

The man perceiving this began to cry out upon my yong Tooth drawer and said that he had spoyled him, the Tooth-drawer seeing his error,and fearing his masters correction : (having a quicke wit) said to the Country man, friend let not my Master know that I did draw you two teeth out, for if he doe,he will make you pay for two; the poore man, fearing his words,to save his purse,paide him for one tooth,and caried the other as secret as though he had stolne it, and the third that pained him,he carried home in his head. Take heed how you draw teeth therefore.

For the falling downe of the Pallat of the mouth.

The cause of it is the recourse of humors from the head to that place,it is knowne by the sight,and great difficulty in swallowing of meate.

Take

Take ſalt well dryed, and pepper beaten, mingle them together and touch the pallat therewith.

A Mouth Water.

Take thrée branches of Roſemary, nine ſage leaves, and twenty Acorne cups; boyle them in a pint of water with one ſpoonefull of honny, and ſo much allome as an haſſell nut, waſh it with this water being well warmed, and it will helpe it, it is alſo good for a ſore throate.

Lay a whole egge that is hard ſodden, (the ſhell being pilled of and the egge bruſed) to the Crowne of the head.

Bakers leaven being layed to the crowne of the head helpeth it.

The Aſhes of Colewort rootes burnt, and put with your thumbe to the pallat, doth help it by drying up of the humors.

For the Cough and hoarſneſſe.

The Cough commeth of ſuperfluous humours that commeth from the head, or of cold, duſt, ſmoake, and ſuch like; hoarſenes is when the humour falleth into the windepipe: for this I will ſet downe ſome few, but good remedies for the poorer ſort, for the rich let them uſe the counſell of the Phyſition, who is to be honored for our healthes ſake.

Séeth Bay berries in water, and receive the fume thereof at your noſtrils and eares, and that will dry up the diſtilling humor.

A good remedy.

Take halfe a pinte of good aqua vitæ, and two ounces of fine ſuggar, ſet them on the fire, and when it beginnes to be hot, ſet fire thereon, and let it ſo burne that it may be like a ſurrup: take thereof morning, and evening, two ſpoonefuls at a time, and you ſhall finde great comfort by it.

Another.

Take muſtard ſéede and beate it groſly, then put it into

blew figges and eate three of them morning and evening, it doth dissolve the grosse humors, and openeth the Conduits of breathing.

Another.

Take Almonds, and blanch them, then stampe them with honny and eate of it, it easeth a long continued Cough.

Some old women, say that a cold Apple eaten to bedward, is good for the Cough. Let them, that have over hot stomackes use it, for my part I know a good Cup of buttered Ale is not amisse, and that is my medicine.

For one that hath suddainely lost his strength, and through debility of the vitall, and naturall spirits, is ready to fall into a Consumption.

This cometh commonly after some great evacuations, as some greate fluxes of the belly, or some vehement motion, also sorrow, feare, and of intemperate, and disordered living; you may know it by faint sweates, and weakenes of all parts interior, and exterior: let the patient eate meate of light disgestion and of good nourishment, and above all things, avoyd anger, and let him use merry, but honest Company.

Let the patient eate every morning two egges, that are reare roasted, and let him mingle with them, white Sugarcandy, nutmegs beaten, and white amber, of each alike; this is very nourishing.

An excellent Drinke for all those that are weake or in a Consumption.

Take two gallons of small Ale, Almonds blanched halfe a pound, Aniseeds, three ounces, foure sticks of good liquerish slyced, red roseleaves, two branches of each: boyle them, till halfe be consumed, then straine them, and adde to it one quarte of good malmsie, drinke thereof, morning and evening, two houres before you eate; this drink preserveth a man

from

from the Cough, makes a man of a strong constitution, and helpeth very much against the Consumption.

An approoved remedy used by a learned German Doctor with great successe.

Take of your garden Snailes, and put them in a bucket with a handfull of salt, and they will scoure themselves, from their slyme, then wash them agayne in fresh water, then boyle them in other water, but not much, but onely, that you may picke them out of their houses; being out of their houses, boyle them in a pottle of new milke so long that they are all to peeces, and the milke thick thereof, then straine them, and adde Sugar-candy that is very white, thrée ounces, foure fat Nutmegs slyced, Cinamon beaten halfe an ounce, sixe dates clensed, and cut very small; boyle all these againe, on a soft fire a little while, and then reserve it to your use, drinke thereof first, and last, and you shall finde great profit by it.

Another good medicen for the same.

Take a good plumpe Cock, put it into a gallon of running water in a close pot that is well covered, adde thereto thrée branches of Rosemary, halfe an ounce of Cinamon, grossly beaten, one ounce of Chyna roote, sixe Cloves, one Nutmegge, a little swéete Margeram, and the bottom of a penny white loafe; boyle these til half be consumed, then take up the Cocke, and let the patient smel thereto, for it will strengthen his spirits, and let him drinke the broath, as he hath a stomacke.

Against fluxes of the Belly.

The fluxes of the Belly, is a disease that weakens a man very much in a short time; it is caused often times by eating of much raw fruite, also by great heate or cold, and chéefly by ulcers in the bowels, by receiving of unproper medicens inward, that are purgative.

Above all things, let the patient take héede of using much

cold

cold drinke, and let him keepe his belly very warme, and not sit long on the close stoole, or other place, where he easeth himselfe

Venice Treakle is good for all fluxes of the belly.

A good and pleasant Medicine.

Take sallet oyle, halfe a pint, of nutmegs beaten halfe an ounce, of Cinamon, one ounce, of mace, a quarter of an ounce, of fine sugar, halfe a pound; mingle these together, and eate of it, three or foure times a day, it hath cured many to my knowledge.

Another.

Take blanched Almonds and boile them in hony till they be blacke, and eate them fasting, it doth restaine the fluxe wonderfully.

Another.

Take old cheese and toast it, and then dry it, and take thereof with Sugar, and it stoppeth very much.

Another.

Take pouder of Comfry rootes and acorne cups, Cinamon grosly beaten, and one Nutmegge slyced; boyle these in a pottle of milke, then straine the milke, and adde foure yolkes of egges to it, and eate thereof every morning, it is exceeding good.

Another.

Take a Slate tyle; burne it, and then pouder it very fine, and mingle it with three yolkes of egs, and bake it in a pan and eate it, this cured one that had it halfe a yeare.

Another secret of worthy esteeme.

Take a pottle of milke, and boyle it in an earthen pot till the th: fourth part be consumed; then have a quarte of plantaine water, and put one pint into it, and so let it boyle, till the fourth part be consumed, then put in the other pint of water and let it boyle as before, till the fourth part be consumed; then reserve it, and drinke thrée times a day thereof, this is a sure and good receite.

Counsell for the Iiske.

Make a board hot, and sit thereon, also apply a hot Trencher to your navill, and it will ease you. Take also of Irish Uate, and drinke it, it is very good.

Of wormes in the Body.

Wormes are engendred divers waies, but chéefly they are bred with putrified phleame, in the Stomacke or Bowels; from this disease procéedeth great paine in the stomacke and Belly, with a great desire of meate: many people die of them, for they bréed sharpe feavers which are dangerous, therefore I will set downe some remedies, such as I know have béene tryed and approved good.

Remedies.

The best and safest way is to take of pure Aloes, beate it to pouder, and take a little in the cold pap of a roasted Apple; this is knowne to be good, and may be given to the weakest people.

Another.

Let the Patient drinke raw milke, foure dayes together, the first day give him garlicke, stamped in Milke to drinke, and put a little suggar therein.

Another.

Take Tansie, and a little Worme-wood, and boyle it in a quarte of water, then straine it, and put hony thereto, and séeth it, and scame it; drinke hereof morning and evening, and it will kill all Wormes whatsoever.

Another.

Boyle scraping of Hartes horne in Milke, and drinke it, and it will helpe you.

Also Garlicke boyled in Milke, is excellent therefore, if the Navell be anoynted with bitter Almonds, and the iuce of Worme-wood, it will kill them.

A Plaster.

Take the iuce of Worme-wood, and a little Oxe gaule, mingle these with a little Wheaten meale, and the white of an egge, and spreade it on a leather, and lay it round about the Navell, it will cause abundance of Wormes to be avoyded.

Another.

Take the iuce of Mint, Ribwort, Orpin, Peachleaves, and houseleeke; mingle these with strong vinegar, Oxe gaule, oyle of Peaches, and Smallidge seede beaten, make an oyntment and use it to the Belly and Navell, or els make it a plaster as was taught before. This is approved.

For the Emeroyds or Piles.

There are certaine veins which end in the fundament, these many times are oppressed with mellancholy blood, so that they are vere painefull and doe oftentimes bleed exceedingly, for this infirmity use some of these remedies that follow.

A good remedy, that is often approoved.

Take three little bagges, made of old linnen cloth, fill them with wheaten meale, let them be of that bignesse, that they may be so great as a goose egge; when that they are filled then put some white wine over a chafing-dish with coales and let the bagges be through hot therein, and apply one to the

the fundament, and when that is cold, take a nother doe this for the space of halfe an houre, morning and evening.

Annoynt the place afterward and lay thereto with a little wooll, oyle of Roses, rubbed in a leaden morter till it be of a leaden Colour.

This hath given many men ease, when divers other things failed, therefore take it as a great secret.

Another.

Take the leaves of henbane, and purslaine, cut them very small, then take crummes of whitebread, and boyle all these in milke, till they be very soft; then put the milke from them, and beate them with the yolke of a hard roasted egge, and oyle of Roses, and apply it to the fundament, it doth helpe the same very speedily.

Another.

Take an Unguent that the Apothecarie calleth populeon, and of the unguent called Album, mingle them together and apply it.

Also the unguent called Pompholigos is very good applyed plasterwise.

Another.

Take Eldern leaves the least, that be tender, and Chickweed, fry these with sweete butter, till that the hearbes are dry, then straine them, and with the liquor that cometh forth anoynt the piles, and dip wooll therein, and apply it.

Another.

If that the piles be swolne and are painefull, yet doe not run, then boyle horehound in water and wine, and salt, put it into a close stoole, and sit over the same, and receive the fume into your body, so hot as you may suffer it, then lay the hearbe so boyled to the fundament.

Another.

Take Mullen, by some called Mullet, the leaves thereof

be hoary, and white; boyle of these leaves in Wine, and bath it with the liquour, and then lay of the leaves to the place, where your paine is, and it helpeth.

For the Stone in the Reines or Bladder.

The Stone is a grievous and pittifull disease, and the poore are much troubled with it, as well as the rich; it proceedeth from great heate, which doth dry up grosse humors into hard Stones, which descend from the kydnies, into the bladder, tormenting the poore Patient with intollerable pain; in this disease the counsell and skill of a learned Physition, is needfull, yet for the comfort of poore people, that cannot alwaies have their good assistance, I will set downe certaine good choyce remedyes, that have helped many.

Remedies for the Stone.

Take nine Iuie berries, dry them, and give them in white Wine warme, it doth mightily provoke urine, and purgeth gravell.

Another.

Take the stones that are found in a Haddocks head, beate them to pouder, and drinke them in white Wine.

The stone cald Oculus Cancri doth the same.

The stones of Medlers poudred doth the like.

The like doth the stone that is found growing in the gall of some Oxen.

Receive this as a great secret.

There is a Beast which lives in the Sea, in the West-Indies, called a Sea-Cow, or Mannatee, this beast or Fish, hath certaine stones that grow in his head; the pouder of this stone drunk in Wine, or other liquour causeth the taker thereof presently to make water and to voyde gravill: many that hath traveld in those parts will affirme this for truth.

A learned Author saith, that if you doe annoynt your yard and

and the share, with the blood of a Fore the stone will breake incontinently, for saith the same Author, put a stone into the blood of a Fore, and it will breake in three dayes.

Another.

Take egge shels dry, them and beate them unto a pouder, it will breake the Stone, it hath beene prooved.

Another.

Boyle seaven heads of Garlike, in raine water, and give the same water to the patient for to drinke, three dayes together, it is prooved for to helpe in this disease.

A Remedy for the Stone strangely found out.

A certaine High Dutchman, being very well skild in cutting for the Stone, was on a time called to an old Gentleman, which was very much troubled with that Infirmity, he having searched him, found the stone to be of such an extraordinary bignesse, that he would not deale with it, a while after this Gentleman dyed, he being acquainted with his friends, desired to open him for to see the stone, in breife he did, and found it so great, and of such a length, and hardnes, that he wondred thereat, for it was so big that he made a haft for a knife thereof; this knife he being once at supper, left on the Table, and the cloath being taken up, the knife was (unwittingly) taken up with it, and so cast on one side with the fragments; next day he missed his knife, and search was made fore it, and it was found in a voyder, amongst scrapings and peeces of Raddish rootes: but so strangely altered that he greatly wondered thereat, for through the vertue of the Radish (against that disease) the haft was found wholly to be consumed: which made him ever after, for to use Radish, against that disease.

Whether this be true or not, I will not examine, but this I know. Take a Radish roote and steepe it in white Wine, all night, and give it to drinke, to one that cannot make his water, it will worke very effectuall, and voyd both water and gravill.

Of the swelling of the Cods.

The swelling of the Cods cometh by outward, and inward occasions, the inward cause is abundance of bad humors, which often times take their course to those parts, much offending the poore patient with great paine; this cure cheifly consisteth in remooving of the cause by phisicall meanes.

The outward cause of this swelling, is taking of great cold, also blowes and strokes; the signes are apparent, great swelling, and rednesse, with extraordinary paine.

A Remedy.

Take one pint of new milke, the crums of white or wheaten Bread, one handfull of Chickweede, one handful of mallowes, chop the hearbes small, and boyle them in the milke: then adde thereto a quarter of a pound of sweete butter, and apply this warme to the part that is pained, and trusse it up with his shirt or napkin, and in short time he shal find ease.

Another Remedy if it be red or inflamed.

Take Beane meale, halfe a pint, sallet oyle, a quarter of a pint, (if you have no oyle, take sweete butter) vinegar a little, mingle all these together, and apply it cold, you shall see it worke effectually, above your expectation.

When the Cods are sweld with much paine.

Take wheaten bran, and the dregges of strong ale, boyle these together and put a peece of sweete butter thereto, and apply it to the part hot. This will give ease without faile.

Another.

Take beane Flower, and mingle it with the iuce of walwort and sweete oyle, apply it to the Cods and it taketh away the swelling incontinent.

Another.

Another.

Take Cow dung and dissolve it in Wine, and fry it with sweet butter, and it taketh away the swelling of the cods.

For Warts, and Cornes.

Warts are of divers formes, and very troublesome, by reason that for the most part, they are on the hands, which are continually used, they procéede of a mellancholly humor, and are cured according to their formes; Corns procéed most commonly from wearing of straite shooes, they are cause of much paine, by reason they doe most commonly, grow on or about the féete.

For the first that are called Warts, if they doe grow in such a forme, that they are lesser at the roote, than at the head, then knit a silke thread about them and every day tye it straiter, at the last it will cut the wart off without bléeding, if you doe wet your thread in Mercury water, it will be the better: if it be bigger at the roote than at the head, then put Brimstone, in pouder thereon and set fire to it, and so burne it out, though this be painefull, yet it is the best way, and wil not suffer them to grow againe.

Remedies for Wartes.

Take the iuce of marrigolds, and wet your wartes therwith, and dry them against the Sunne, do this thrée or foure times, and it will cure them.

Another.

Take a red Snaile and bruse it with salt, and take the iuce and wet the wartes with it, and it will kill them.

Another.

Take -wartwort, or spurge, and wet them with the iuice, and it will heale them.

Purslaine

Purslaine rubbed on the Warts consumeth them.

Remedies for Cornes.

The best way is to cut them so deepe as you can. But it were best to tye a little peece of veale, all the night on the Corne, and cut it in the morning.

After that you have cut the Corne fill up the hole with the sand that growes on the bottom of a foule chamber pot, and over it lay a plaster of red waxe.

Another

Take a Cowes gaule, and wet it therewith, and it will plucke it up by the rootes.

Another.

Take of the powder of Aristabours, and mingle it with Barrowes grease, and it will make it fall in foure dayes, then put Copperice into the hole.

For the Gout.

The Gout is caused as the Phisitions hold opinion, by excesse, as surfetting, drunkennesse, much using of Womens company, immoderate exercise, and also by much ease; the doctors know better how to give names to it than to cure it, for a Welchman hath not more names (and harder) than it hath; as for example, they call it Sciatica, Chiragra, Podagra, pechiagra, Gonagra, and Arthritica; it commonly keepes good company, as Bishops, Cardinals, Dukes, Earles, Lords, Knights, Judges, Gentlemen, and Merchants; the reason is (as it is thought) for the bad entertainement that it once had, at a poore mans house, when master Gout was a traveller, which a witty, and well conceited Author sets downe in this manner.

A tale that is true enough.

A great while agoe, when Monsieur Gout was not so rich (as now he is;) he was forced to travell, as other poore men are sometime, in his travel he met with a spider, whose journey lay as Mr. Goutes did: they being both benighted, they sought lodging, and came to a poore mans house, which the Gout tooke up for his lodging, for he being alwayes a laisie companion, would goe no farther, but the Spider being more nimble, went to a rich mans house, and there tooke up his lodging for that night: the next day they met againe, and asked each other of their entertainement the passed night, mine saide the Gout, was the worst as ever I had, for I had no sooner touched the poore mans legs, thinking ther to take my rest, but up he gets, and to threashing he goes, so that I had no rest the whole night. And I, saide the Spider, had no sooner begun to build my house, in the rich mans chamber, but the Mayde came with a broome, and tore downe all my worke, and so fiercely did pursue me, that I had so much adoe to save my life, as ever I had.

Seeing it is so then, saide the Gout, we will change lodging, I will goe to the rich mans house, and thou shalt goe to the poore mans: they both were well content, and did so, and found such ease and rest in their lodging, that they resolved never to remoove, for the Spider builded and was not troubled, the Gout he was entertained with a soaft Cushion, with downe Pillowes, with dainty Caudels, and delicate broathes; in briefe: he did like it so well, that ever since he takes up his lodging with rich men, where I desire that he should take his rest, rather than in my poore house.

Then may one say, if that poore men be free of it, what neede I to speake thereof? I doe it for poore prodigals, who often spend their monies, yet keepe this disease.

Remedies to ease the Gout.

Take the fat of a Cat, Goose grease, Badgers grease, Fox

grease, of each alike; then take Ivy, Sage, Bay leaves, Rosemary, White Wax, yolkes of roasted egges, with a quantity of red Snailes: bruse them together & them put into a pot that hath holes made in the bottome for that purpose, and let it be close covered that no ayre may issue forth: put under this pot another that is whole, and bury them into the earth, so farre as the mouth of the uppermost pot, then make a good fire thereupon, and you shall have in the bottome of the lowermost pot a precious oyntment that is good for the Gout.

Another.

Take Tyme, and the white of an egge, beate them together, and apply it plasterwise and it is both a good and healthfull medicen for the Gout.

Another.

Take Hares dung, mingle it with wine and apply it warme, and it healeth those that are pained with the Gout.

Another.

Use a bath of Sea water, and it will ease you.

Also a bath wherein Dock-leaves, and Emmets with their egges have beene sodden, doth the like.

Another.

Take Wormewood, Walwort, Wheate bran, Goates dunge; boyle them in vinegar till the vinegar be consumed, then stampe it and apply it hot.

For all manner of Burning whether it be with fire, pouder, lead, oyle, or any other thing.

Divers times it happens, that Men, Women, and Children, come to strange mishaps by burning and scalding, and the friends, and parents of the parties so burnt (by reason of their remote dwelling, and want of skill in such casualties) are

are not furnished with such remedies as are to be used in such accidents, for the releefe of them onely, I have set downe such things as are both good, and easy to be gotten uppon such occasion, you may be bold to use them, for I know them safe and sure.

For burning with common Fire.

Take fresh butter and melt it, then poure it into cold water, and wash it so long that it be so white as snow; then poure the water off, and reserve the butter in a pot, with this only dresse the burning, and it shall fetch al the fire out; that being done, heale it with some skinning salue, as you shall find in the booke.

Whether it be oyle, milke, or water, wherewith the patient is scalded withall, you neede use no other thing to fetch the fire out but this.

For burning with Iron, Lead, Copper, or any other mettle.

If the burning be with any mettle, as Iron, Lead, or such like, then shall you not presently apply fat things to it, but do as I shal direct you, and you shall be sure to find benefit by it.

Take nightshade water, and snow water, mingled, and apply it to the burning with linnen cloath doe this 24. houres together, in which time the fire will be out of it; then do this.

Take fat Bacon, cut it in small peeces, and melt it then poure it into snow water, and beate it that it be very white, then apply it thicke to the burning, and you shall finde, that it will doe what you did expect.

When the fire is out, use some skinning plaster, these things are plaine, but sure. yet to give full satisfaction to all, I will set downe some other things that are approoved.

Remedies.

Take oyle of nuts, and common Wax, melt them together and use it.

Lintseed oyle, or common oyle will doe the like.

Another.

Take Lime, and wash it in nine severall waters, then mingle it with common oyle, but stirre it exceedingly; with this annoynt the place, and it will helpe it.

Another.

Take the white of an egge, and mingle it with oyle of Roses, or common oyle, till it becom an oyntment; apply it with cloth thereto, and it will heale without any great or manifest scarre.

Another.

If the skin be not broken, then stampe Onions with salt, and apply it with linnen cloath.

Or use blacke soape, or honny mingled, and it will keepe it from blistering, but take heede that you use it not where that the skinne is broken, for it will cause great paine.

Another.

Take butter milke, wet cloathes therein, and apply it to the burning, and it will take the fire out of it; also cheese curdes will doe the like.

Of the small Pockes, and Measels.

The small Pockes, and measels is common in England, and other Countries, and therefore they neede no description; yet for the furtherance of ignorant people, I will in few words set downe, how that you may know when one is infected, and also what is best to be done in this disease.

Signes.

The signes when one is infected are these, first he, or shee is taken with a hot feaver, great paine in the back, stopping of the nose, beating of the heart, hoarsenes, rednesse of the Eyes, with paine and heavinesse in the head pricking in the whole body, drynesse in the mouth, shortnes of the breath and difficulty in breathing

Good Signes.

When they doe soone and in short time appeare, and that in their comming forth, they doe looke red, and after that they come forth, they doe looke white, and with speed they doe come to ripen; when they do draw the breath easily, and that the Feaver doth leave them, these are good signes.

Ill Signes.

When the Pockes lye hidden in the flesh, and do not come forth, or if after their comming, they doe suddainly strike in againe, and vanish away, or that they doe looke of a black blewish, or greene, colour, that the sicke doe often swound, if their breath is drawne with paine, if he have a great scouring, if that the pockes come double, that is, one growing within another, or when they doe rise like blisters, and suddainely fall flat with a hard blacke crust, as if it had beene burned, all these are ill signes, and death most commonly doth follow them.

The Cure.

For the Cure hereof, you must first strengthen the inward parts and drive the disease outward, and then have a care that both inward and outward, parts be not hurt thereby.

To drive them forth, keepe the sicke body in a reasonable heate, and give unto him the weight of sixe pence of good Treacle in Burrage water.

Or take a quart of posset ale, a handfull of Fennell seede, boyle them till a third part be consumed, then straine it, and put thereto sixpence weight of Treakle, and a little Saffran, give of it to drinke, morning and evening, halfe a pint at a time.

Or take a quarte of ale, put thereto Rosemary, and sweete Margeron, and Sage, with three Bay leaves and a little saffran; boyle them all and drinke thereof a little, and sweate if you can.

Also Saffran boyled in milke, is very good to drinke hot, I have knowne good women use this to their Children, with good successe.

To preserve the Eyes.

Take Rosewater, six spoonefull, Womans milke, that

gives a boy sucke, thrée spoonefull, Sugar candy a little mixt together; apply it to the eyes, with a thrée double cloath till the danger be past.

To preserve the Eares.

Put a drop of oyle of Roses, warme into them ere that he sweate.

To preserve the Nostrils.

Let him smel to red rose vinegar, or boyled with saunders.

To preserve the Throate.

Let him hold alwaies white Sugar Candy in his mouth, and as it melteth, swallow it downe.

To preserve the Lungs.

Give him to drinke Barly water, wherein Liquerish hath béene boyled.

A Salve for them after they are come forth.

When that they are come forth and begin to grow white, then take a pinne, and open them on the top and thrust out the matter inclosed very gently, for it is that matter that by its sharpenesse, eates into the flesh, and leaves such pits as you shall often sée in the faces of those that have had the smal Pockes; when you have done thus, then annoint the places with this oyntment following.

An oyntment for the Pockes.

Take Eldernleaves, one handfull, Marigolds two handfull, French Mallowes, one handfull, Hogs grease, halfe a pound, bruse them and boyle them till they be crisp, then straine it and kéepe it to your use.

If you annoynt them with the oyle of swéete Almonds, it healeth them very faire.

Some use in the sommer time, to touch them every day with the iuce of Marigolds, and so healeth them.

For

For spots in the face when that they are well.

Take iuce of Lemons, and mixe it with bay salt, and touch the spots therewith often times in the day, for it is excellent good.

How to open the Eye-lids, that are fastned together with the Pockes.

Boyle Quince-seedes and Mallowes in faire water, wet double cloathes therein and lay them over the Eyes, continue this till you can open them, and then if you perceive any web or filme to be growne over the sight, put white Sugar Candy poudered into it, or you may dissolue it in Rosewater.

Directions

Directions to the plaine, and honest man, whereby he may know, and truely Iudge, how a person being found dead, came by his end, very fitting to be knowne of such as are called to be Iurers upon Life and Death.

To know whether a person (being found) dead, be killed by Thunder or not.

If it shall happen, that thou art called to give thy Judgement, of a person being found dead, whether he were killed by thunder or lightning, or else came by his death some other way; by these signes following, thou maist truly give thy Judgement thereof.

That person that is killed by thunder, or lightning, his body giveth an evill and strong sulphurous smell, it is of that strength, that it is noysome to all Creatures: for neither beast nor fowle will come neere it, much lesse feede thereon; that part of the body, that is strikẽ, is usually without wound, yet often shall you finde, that the bones of the part are broken; if there be a wound, in the touching thereof you shall find that part where the wound is, farre more colder than any other part of the body, as Pliny witnesseth lib. 2. chap. 34. the reason is, the spirits (being touched most subtilly, by a more subtill and violent winde) are dispersed abroad: this strange wind the thunder and lightning, alwayes driveth before it.

Also the lightning leaveth behinde a signe of burning, by reason it is never without fire, wherewith it burneth those things it toucheth, or makes them blacke.

All beasts that are strucke with thunder or lightning, fall on the contrary side, that they are strucken on.

And

And it is obserbed by the ancient writers, that no man dieth of this stroke unlesse he fall on the same side that he is strucken.

Those that are thunder-strucken sleeping, their eyes continue open, and they that are strucken waking they continue their eyes shut.

Phillip Com: writeth that those bodies that are strucke with thunder or lightning, and die thereof, those bodies are not subiect to rotting, as other bodies are; therefore in old time those bodies were neither burned, nor buried, for as the salt preserves all dead bodies from rotting, so the sulphur that the lightning bringeth with it, keepes the bodies from putrifaction, by reason of his firie and drying heate, which is contrary to all rottennesse, and putrifaction.

To know whether one dyed of the Plague or not.

Those that die of the visitation of God, called commonly the Plague, the corps of such persons, are not so stiffe as those are that die of other sicknesses; the reason of which is this: whiles that the person lived the body was corrupted, and filled with rotten humors, which the sicknesse did engender; but being dead, they spread themselves over the whole corps, for then the putrifaction cometh to its full hight, for there is not then any part which is not filled with a stinking, and rotten Corruption.

Also the bodies of them that die of this sickenesse will presently stinke.

Likewise there sheweth soone after their deathes, some swelling in their groynes, behinde the eares, or else under the Arme pits.

If there appeare no swelling, then you shall perceive small spots in the flesh called by us God Tokens, which spottes, whilst that the sicke lived, lay hidden in the flesh, but being dead, they appeare plaine to the beholders.

Likewise the colour of the nose, the eares, naples, and the whole body is blacker, than those that die of other sicknesse; oftentimes the face likewise is so deformed that their familiar

liar friends can hardly know them.

How to know whether, one were wounded, hanged, or drowned, after they were dead.

If a body be found dead, and with wounds, and you would know whether he or shee, received them living or not, then consider this.

If the body were wounded living, then the wound will be red and bloody, and the lips of the wound will be of a leadish colour and swelled.

But if that he were wounded, after that he was dead; then shall the wound be neither red, bloody, swelled, nor of a leadish colour; by reason that in a dead body all the actions of nature ceaseth, and no blood, nor any living spirit can then be sent toward the wounde.

So also if a man be hanged, whilest that he lived, then shall the Circle of the rope, about his necke, shew of a red and blewish colour, and the skin above it will be rumpled.

The second bone in the necke, will be out of Joynt.

The Armes, face, and legs, will be swelled, and of a leadish colour.

Also you shall finde spittle in his mouth; and snot in his nostrils.

Commonly his breeches are pissed, and his ordure will sticke in his fundament, which commeth with the striving, when he is strangled.

Now in any person, that is hanged after he is dead, there is no such signe; for, as I saide before, the actions of nature ceaseth in a dead man.

And if a person be found dead in the water, and you would know whether he were throwne in alive, or after that he was dead, consider these signes.

The man that is drowned, his stomacke, and belly will be full of water.

Also out of his nose will come a snotty substance, and out of his mouth a scumme, like spittle.

Commonly,

Commonly they will bleede at the nose.

Also the skin will be rubbed off, from his forehead, and fingers ends, by reason of his scrabling at his death to save himselfe.

Now if a body be throwne in, after that he is dead: there is no such signe, for then his Conduits are stopped, and it is impossible for him to have water in his belly: or snot in his nostrils, spittle in his mouth, or any other signe that was shewed before.

The reason of the bodies swimming on the water is the hollownes thereof, which being filled with winde it swimmeth on the water as a blowne bladder will doe.

And these signes, will suffice to instruct any ordinary apprehension.

Now followeth, certaine approoved Remedies, and good Plasters.

For a weake Backe.

Take a quart of milke; boyle therein rosemary flowers, or tops, one handfull.

Cinamon grosly beaten, Cloves, and Mace, of each a little, one Nutmeg sliced, two Dates.

Straine it and adde thereto, one yolke of an egge, a little hony, the pouder of Comfry rootes, and the pouder of acorne tops, drinke thereof morning and at night a good draught.

To make a good, and comfortable drinke.

Take claret or white Wine that is very good, nine pints; of Cinamon, one ounce and a halfe, Sugar, one pound, Gingar, halfe an ounce, Nutmegs, halfe an ounce; beate all these somwhat grosse, and let them stand three daies in the Wine, being close stopped.

Then straine it, and keepe it to your use, it is good for the heating, and comforting, of a cold stomacke.

For a Spraine in the Arme, or Legge.

Take the inward Rinde of the Elderne, boyle it in white

Wine to a good thicknes, and apply it warme, and it will ease you without faile.

For the Ague, it hath holpen many.

Take Hearbe grace, or Rew: beate it with Bay salt, and lay it to the lower spondill of the necke.

A speciall Remedy, for cold, hard and windy swellings.

Take blacke sope, one pound, Barrowes grease, or Bores grease, one pound, aqua vitæ one pinte.

Melt your Barrowes grease and soape, and put to the halfe of your aqua vitæ, then boyle it till the aqua vitæ be consumed, then adde the rest.

A good Sparadrap plaster:

Take common oyle one quart, red lead, and white lead, of each halfe a pound, waxe a quarter of a pound, boyle it till it be blacke, in the cooling, put some duckes grease into it, and dip your cloath therein,

For an Inflammation, it is well approoved.

Take Barly meale, a little bolearmanacke, oyle of Roses, and the white of an egge, mingle these with a little wine vinegar, and apply it cold.

A good greene plaster.

Take wax, turpentine, rosen, of each foure ounces, oyle halfe a pint, frankensence, and masticke halfe an ounce, verdigrease the fourth part of one ounce, and make a Plaster.

A good Red salue that is skinning.

Take Oyle of Roses one pint, white waxe, two ounces, Minium, three ounces, Ceruse, an ounce and an halfe, Tutty, and Camphor, three drams, mingle them well.

A good white plaster.

Take oyle two pound, Ceruse one pound and a halfe, white

white waxe foure ounces, boyle it and make it in Rowles.

This is good for all wringens, or gaules, of the feete, hands, or other parts, it skinneth old ulcers, and is good to cure burnings.

A good water for Itching scabs, and salt Phlegme.

Take of Roch allome, one part, of salt Peter, two parts, boyle them in a pint of vinegar, till halfe be consumed, and use it to the part that is grieved.

An excellent plaster for the wormes, the like thereof hath not beene knowne in *England*.

Take the pouder of earth-wormes, halfe a quarter of an ounce, Coliquintida, Worme seede, Southernwood, and Tansy, take of each of these in pouder halfe, a quarter of an ounce, of Aloes the weight of sixe pence, of Mirre, the weight of three pence; oyle, wormewood, and the gaull of a Bull, as much as will bring the rest into a body; stir them together, in a hot morter, with a hot pestill, till all be well mingled, then use this plaster, in this manner, make two plasters hereof, and the second day, apply a plaster thereof to the mouth of the stomacke.

The third day apply a plaster to the Navill, and the next day give the patient, honny and Milke to drinke, and the wormes, will be killed without faile, this is a great secret, and never yet published in English.

A strange Cure done, by a poore man with little cost, yet with great expedition.

A rich man in the Country, had in one of his legges an extraordinary great swelling, with rednesse, and great paine; it held the part from the Ancle to the knee, so that this rich man could not rest; he spared no cost, yet found no comfort, in all the medicens that were applyed. It chanced that a poore man, (I thinke some Chirurgion) passed that way, and hearing thereof, did intreate that he might sée it, which he did and under tooke to cure it, which he performed in this manner.

He tooke thée iuice of Marigoldes, and a little vinegar, and annoynted all his legge, then dipped he a cloath in the same, and dressed it twise a day, and the third day it was well, to the wonder of those which had formerly séene it.

An excellent salve, and easy to make, fitting for every Countrey man to have in his house.

Take Worme-wood, Smallidge, and large Plantaine, of each alike, adde thereto of Bettonny, as much as halfe of them all; chop these very small, and then beate them, with Deares suet, and Butter, without salt; set them by nine dayes, till they be mouldy; then boyle them till that the hearbes be parched. Then straine them, and put to the strayned liquor white waxe, and a little turpentine, if you have it, then melt it againe, and reserve it to your use.

This is good for all bruses of the legges or Armes, for all spraines or wrenches; for all woundes, whether they be made with sword, or staffe, or any other thing; the use of it will shew its vertues.

What is written in this booke, is written to the poore, and plaine man, not for the rich or learned; nor to instruct gadding women, that they might leave their callings, and turne Chirurgions, to the destruction of many poore men: to none of these purposes, was this published, but for an instruction, for poore householders to help their Children, and Servants in their néede. Vale.

FINIS.